Pancreas Diet 2

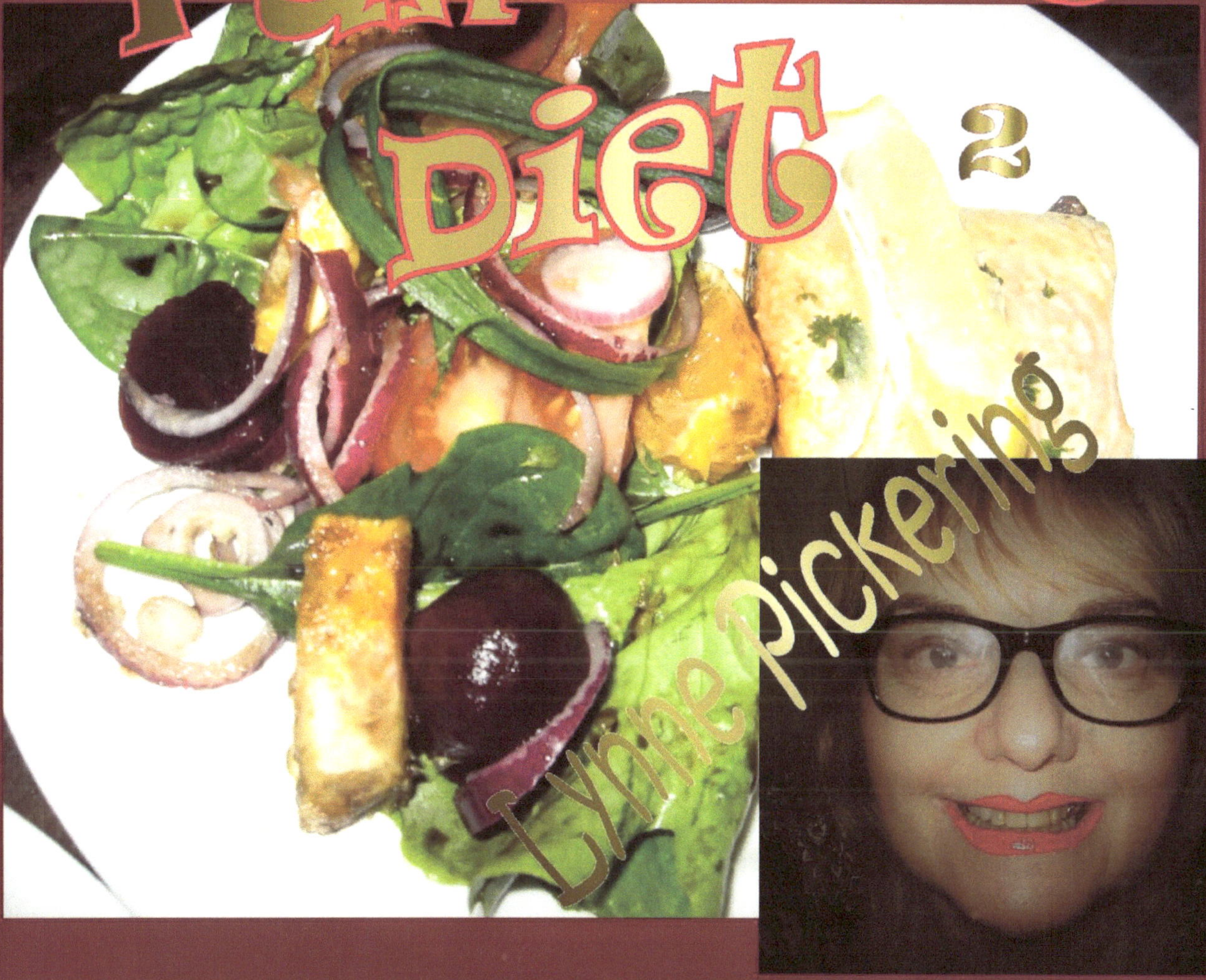

Lynne Pickering

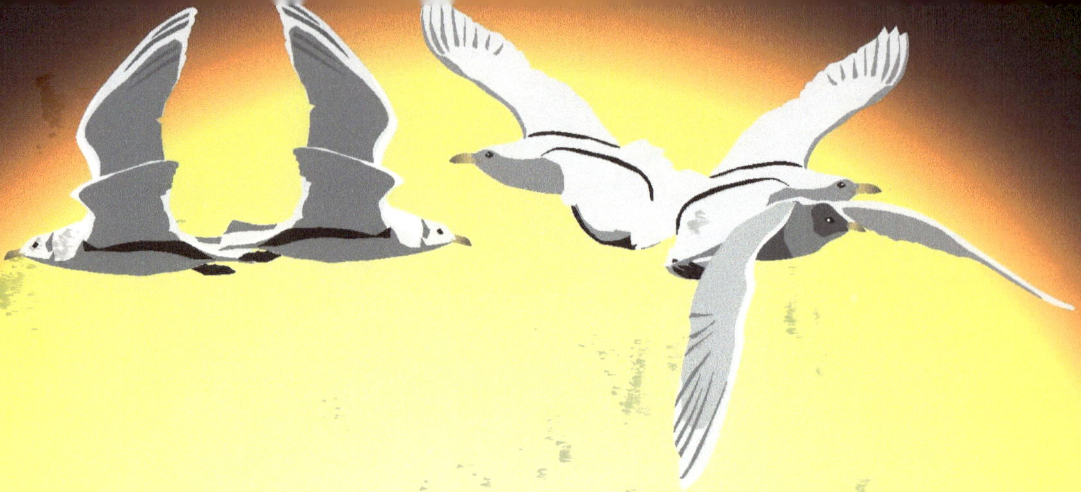

Copyright
Lynne Pickering
Copyright © 2019 Lynne Pickering

ISBN   978-1606481083

All rights reserved. No part of this book may be reproduced or transmitted in any Form or by any means, electronic or mechanical, including photocopying, Recording, or by any information, storage, and retrieval system, without permission in writing from the copyright owner.
This is a work of fiction. Names characters, places and incidents either are the product of the authors imagination
Or are used fictitiously, and any resemblance to any actual persons. Living or dead, events ,or locales is entirely coincidental.

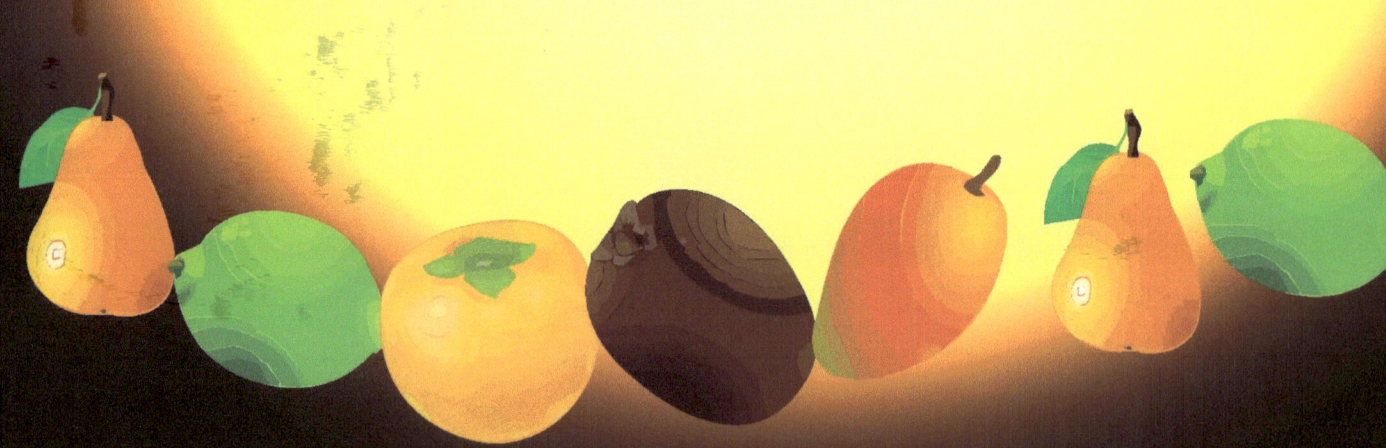

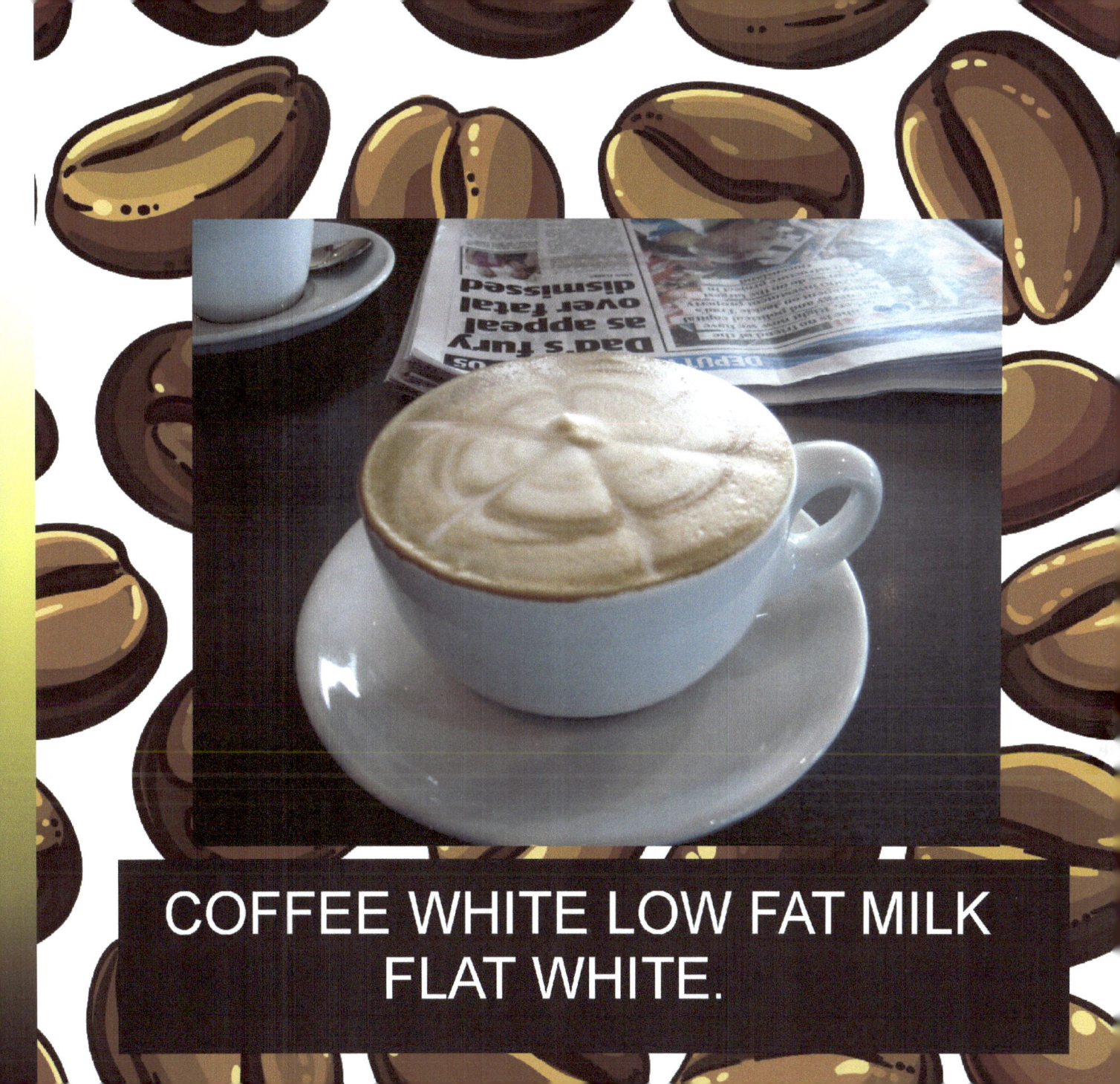

Red salmon cooked in coconut water.

Red salmon cook in 1/2" coconut water in small electric frypan.

Sweet potato mashed no additives.

Cauliflower with green beans steamed

A simple nutricious meal.

Add lemon slice.

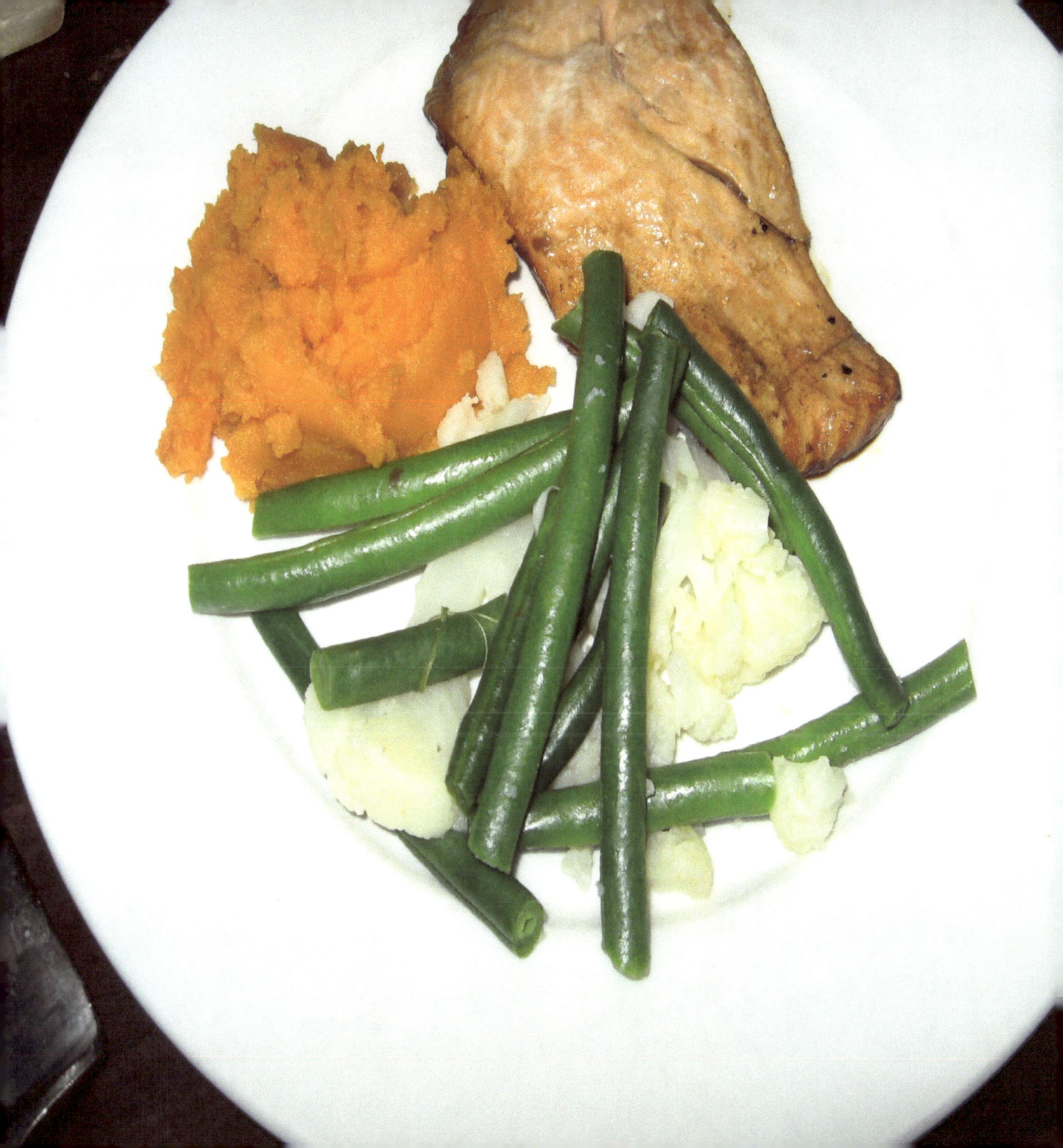

Tropical salad serve with fish

One cup of baby spinich leaves
one orange cut into small squares
One half cup of baby beetroot tinned no sugar
pumpkin seed two table spoons
squeeze half a lemon
One tree ripened tomato
one red onion sliced finley
drizzle Balsamic vinegar over and serve.

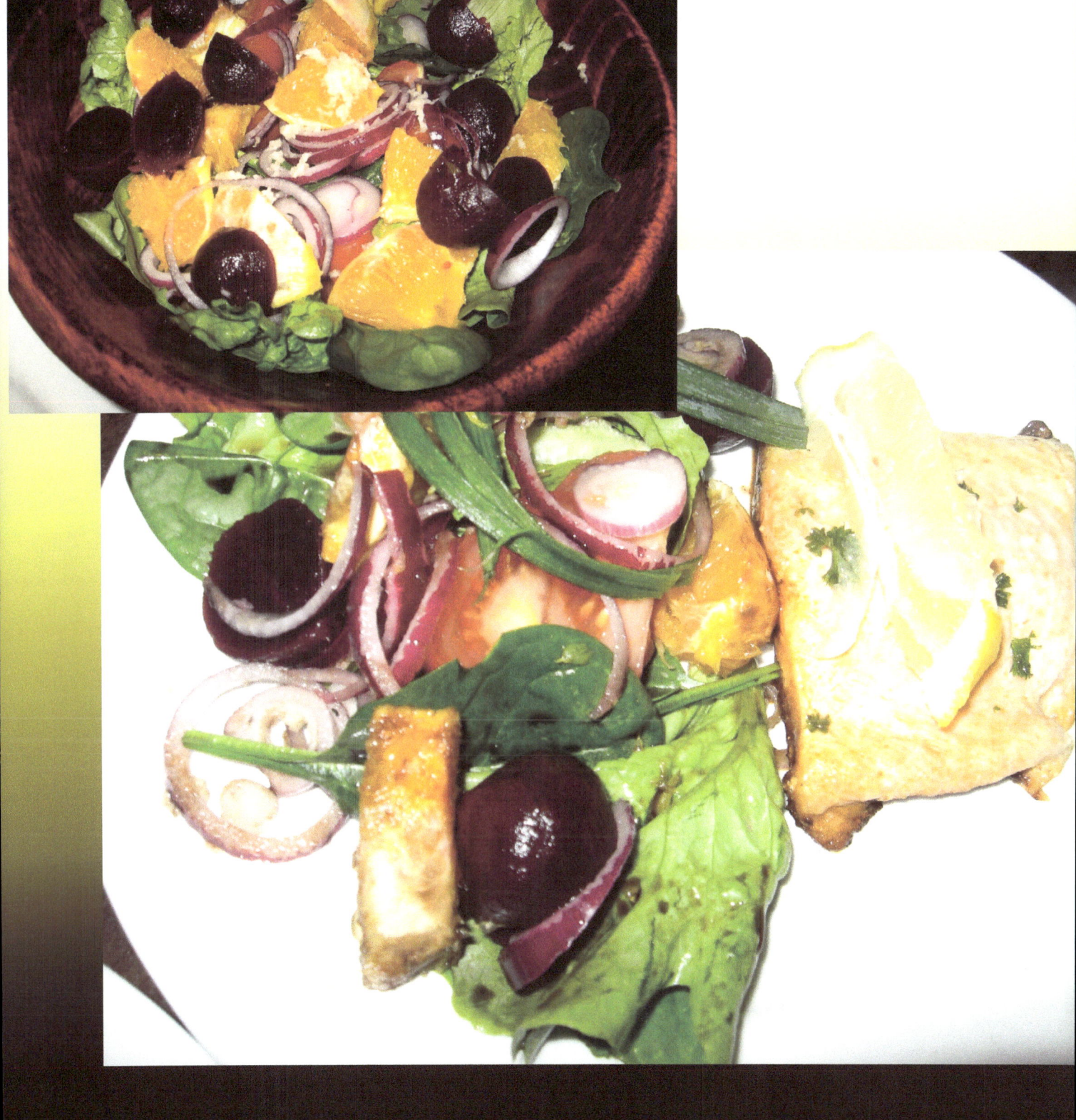

Tuna and sweetorn mornay

3 cups low fat milk.
thicken with 2 tablespoons cornflour
add 1 tin drained sweet corn whol kernals
one medium time tuna drain in spring water (drain of water)
2 tablespoons of sliced shallots
One shake of basil leaves about 1/2 teaspoon.
Bring slowly to a simmer in an electric skillet pan.

Tuna & Sweetcorn Mornay

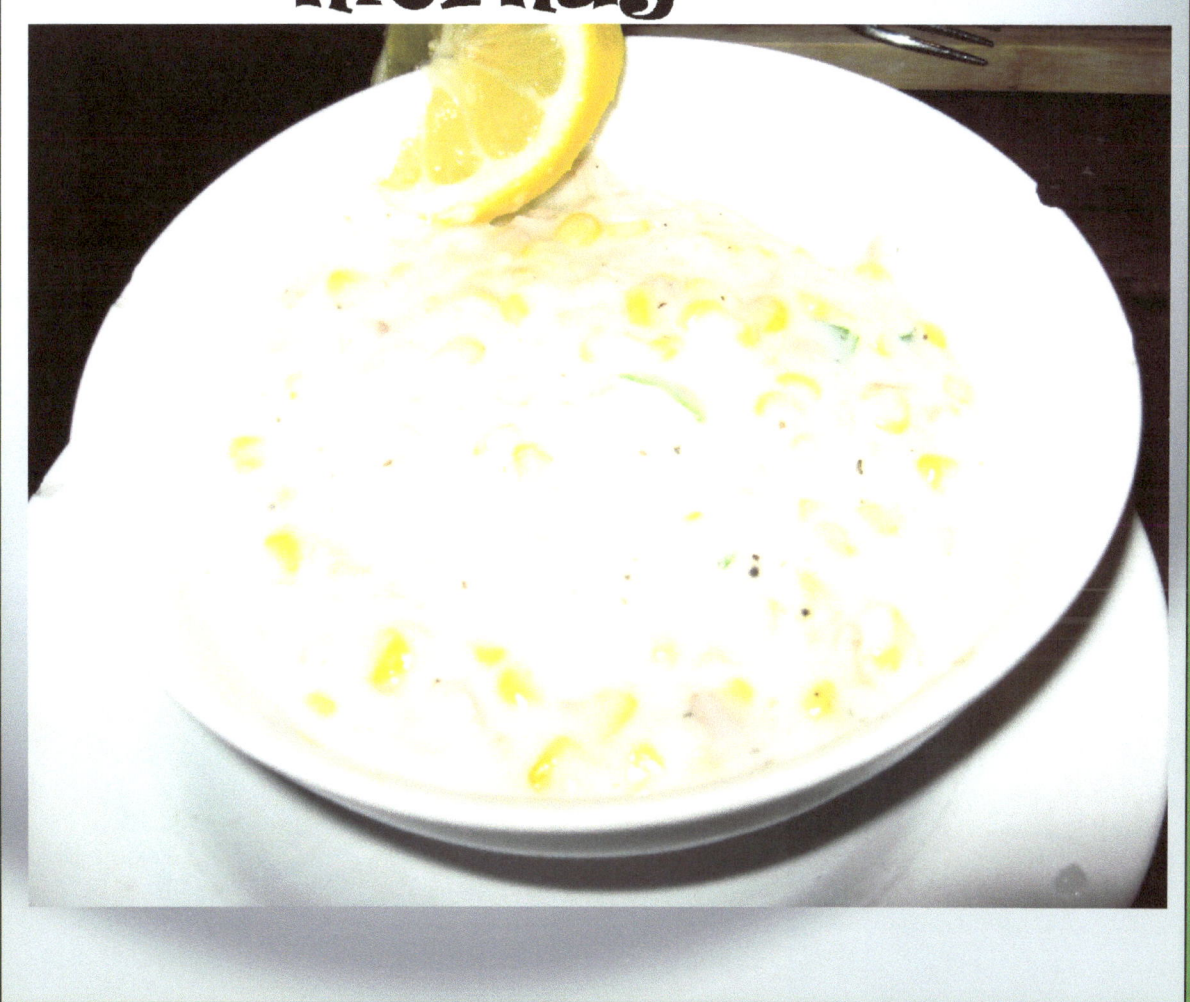

Coconut Chicken Mornay

4 pieces fresh skinned chicken fillets
One Head Broccoli
one carrot cut into straws
6 small mushrooms sliced
2 cups chicken stock
half tin light coconut milk

In small electric pan cut chicken into small pieces cook in a small amount of chicken stock fill pan.
Add carrot, sliced mushrooms.broccili when cooked add in the last two minutes coconut light milk
serve on steamed rice.

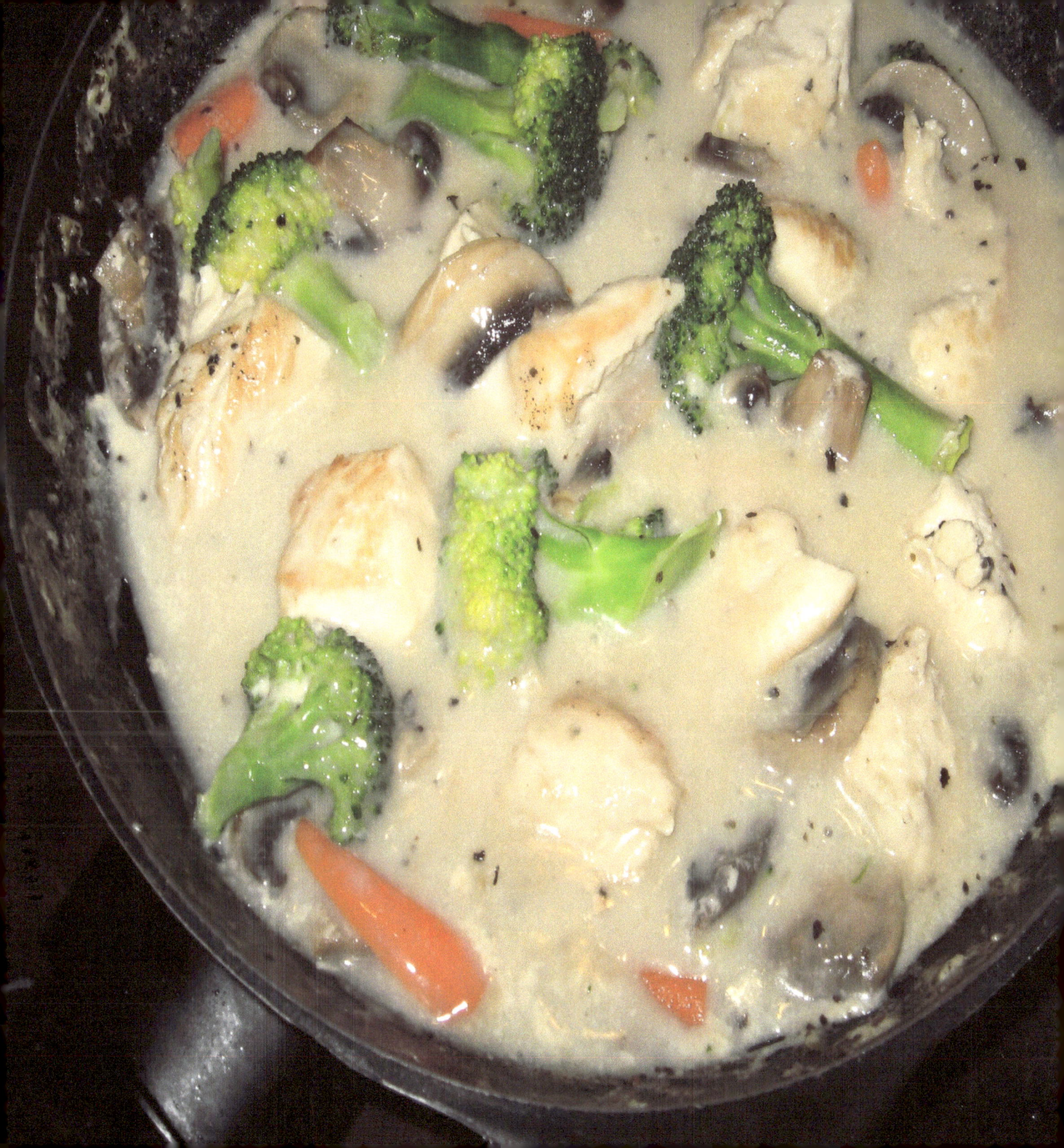

Lunch Special Salad and boiled egg.

Lettuce exotic
sweet potato grilled diced squares
Spanish onion sliced.
small tomatos on vine about 5
sliced cucumber small
sprinkle of basil

Boiled egg 4 minutes so soft inside.
Sprinkle French salad dressing over salad.

Serve with egg.

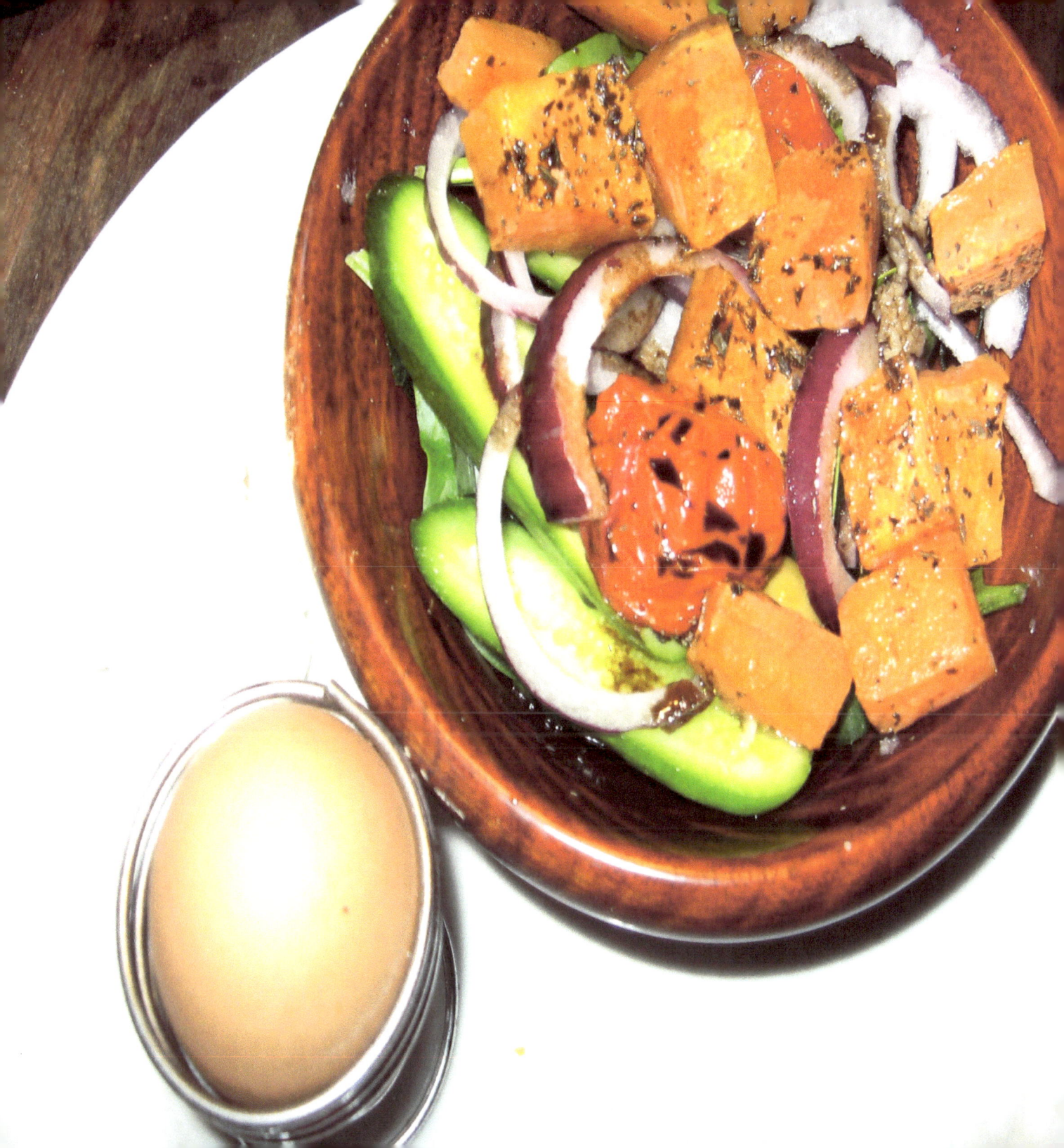

Thai red chicken

SERVES 2

3 Jalapenos (small mild chilli)
4 pieces of chicken tenderloins
1/2 head broccili, 1/3 cup shallots
1/3 cup sliced finely celery
1 tablespoon Thai Red curry paste
1 cup champiogions button mushrooms
2 cups chicken broth (no addiditives)
Serve on Jasmine steamed rice.
COOK CHICKE IN SMALL PIECES IN CHICKEN STOCK IN SMALL FRYPAN ADD Thai red curry and mushrooms , Jalapenos cut finely add broccili last two minutes before serving.

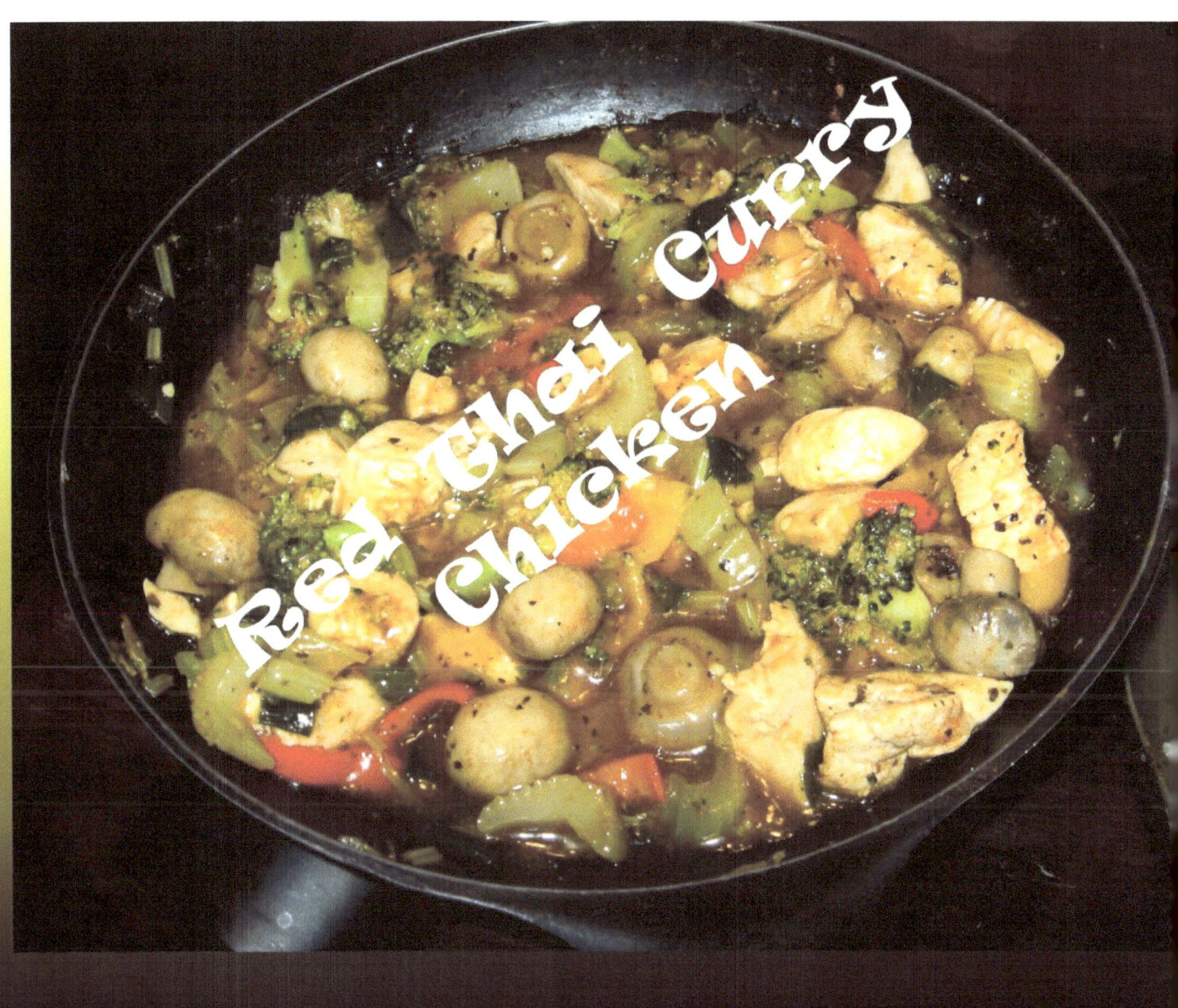

SALMON OMELETTE

4 EGGS BREATEN WITH WHISK
SMALL AMOUNT OF COCONUT OIL
POUR INTO PAN
ADD STRIPE OF COTTAGE CHEESE
SPRINKLE DICED SHALLOTS
1/3 CAPSICAN COPPED INTO SQUARES
SMALL TIN SALMON SPREAD OVER OMELETTE
TINY VINE TOMATOES 4 CUT IN HALF

FOLD OMELETTE SERVE COOK
ONLY ONE SIDE.

ENJOY

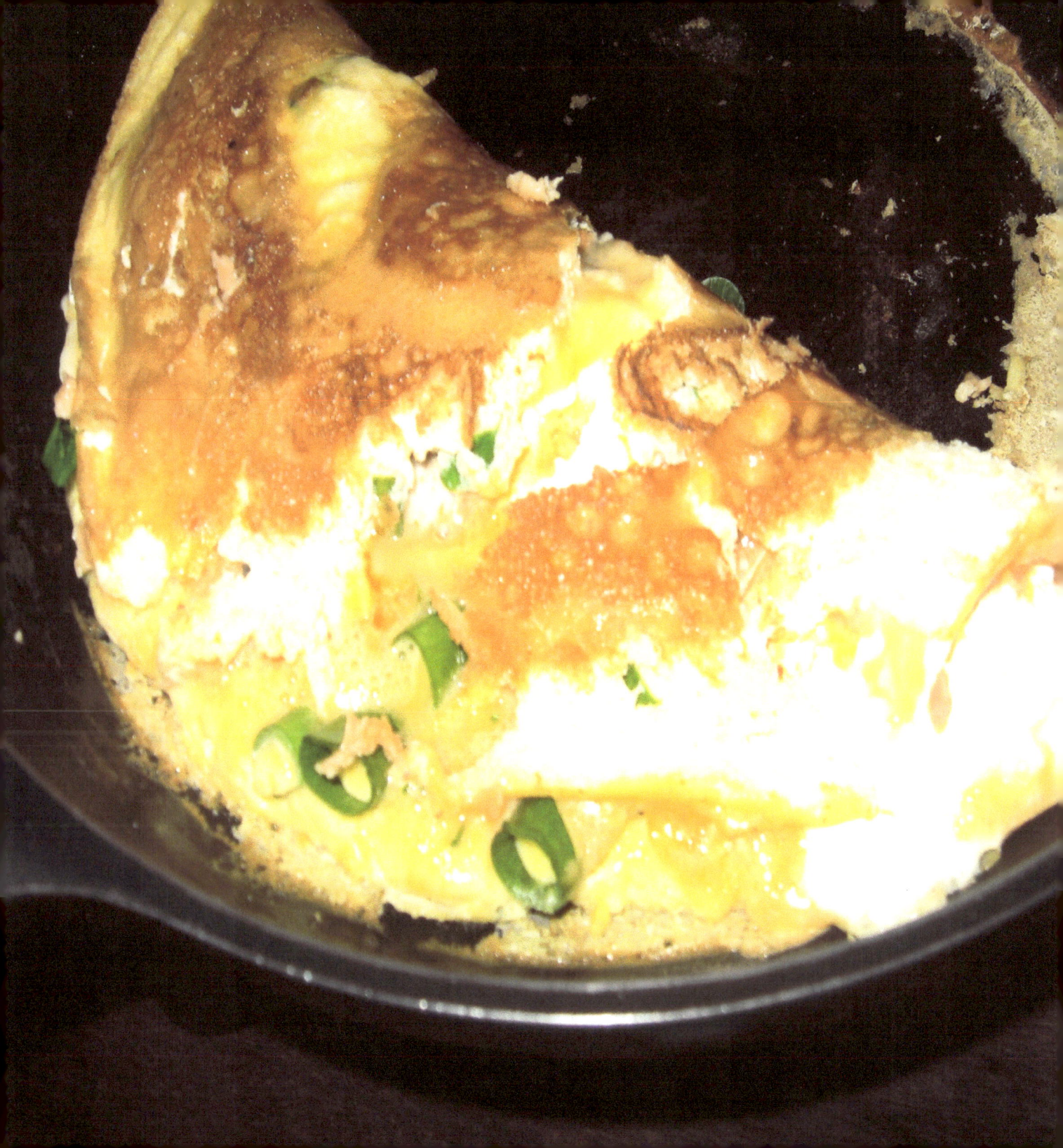

CHICKEN AND CABBAGE STIR FRY

4 SMALL SKINNED BREASTS OF CHICKEN
ONE CARROT
1/2 SMALL SUGARLOAF CABBAGE
SHALLOTS CHOPPED
MUSHROOMS ABOUT 4 SLICED
COCONUT WATER TWO CUPS.
COOK IN SMALL FRYPAN SERVES TWO.
ADD SALT FREE SOYA SAUCE 1 TABLESPOON

SERVE ON STEAMED RICE.

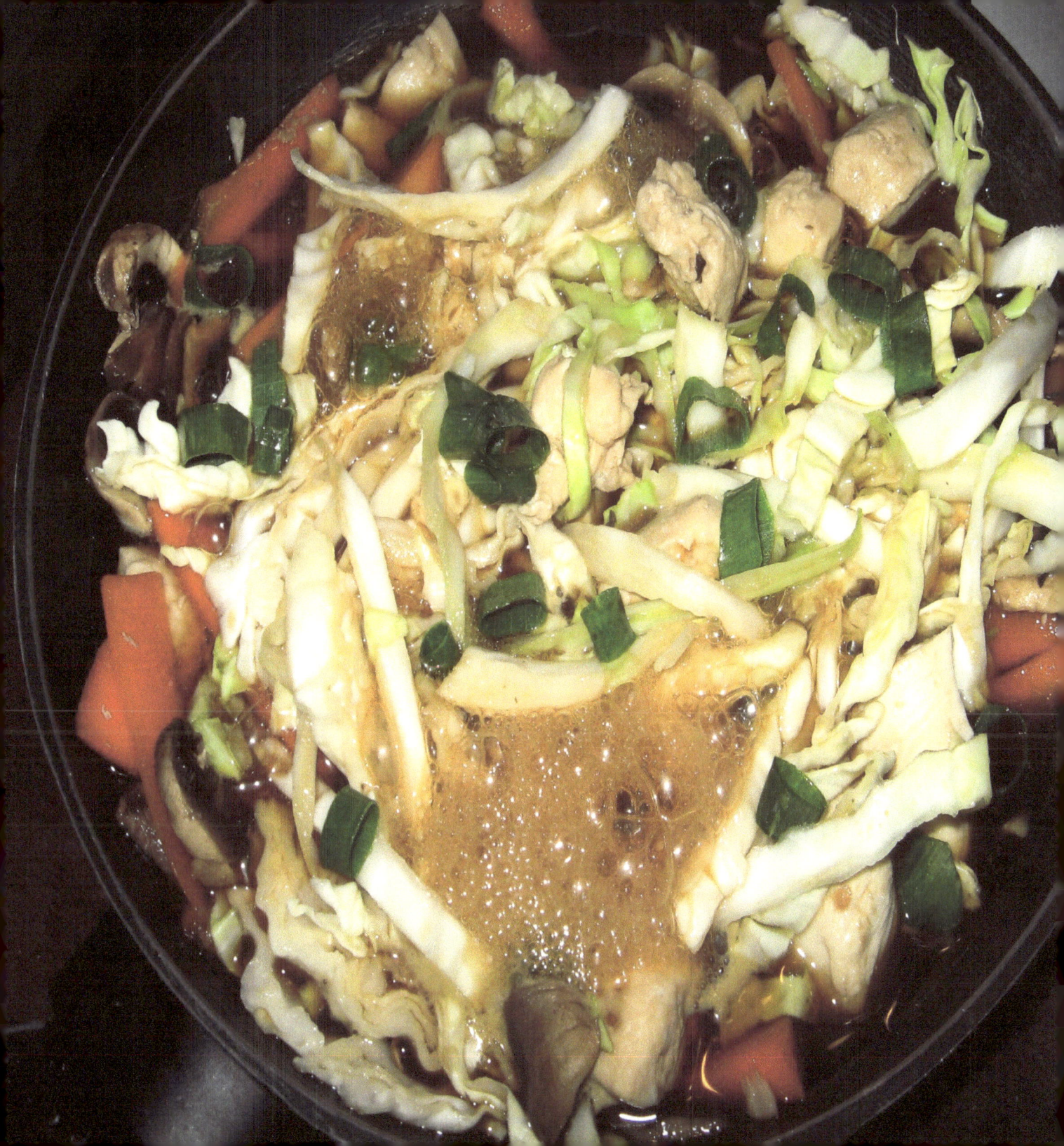

Chicken stir fry with Tumeric.

4 small fillets of chicken skinned
2 cups coconut water
1 carrot cut into slices
2 tablespoons of CLIVE OF INDIA
or tumeric and lemon grass
1 soup spoon of cranberries
1 spoonful of raisons
10 snow peas
sliced small cucumber

cook chicken diced into small pieces
add all ingrediants except snow peas
ass at last moment.
Serve on steamed rice.

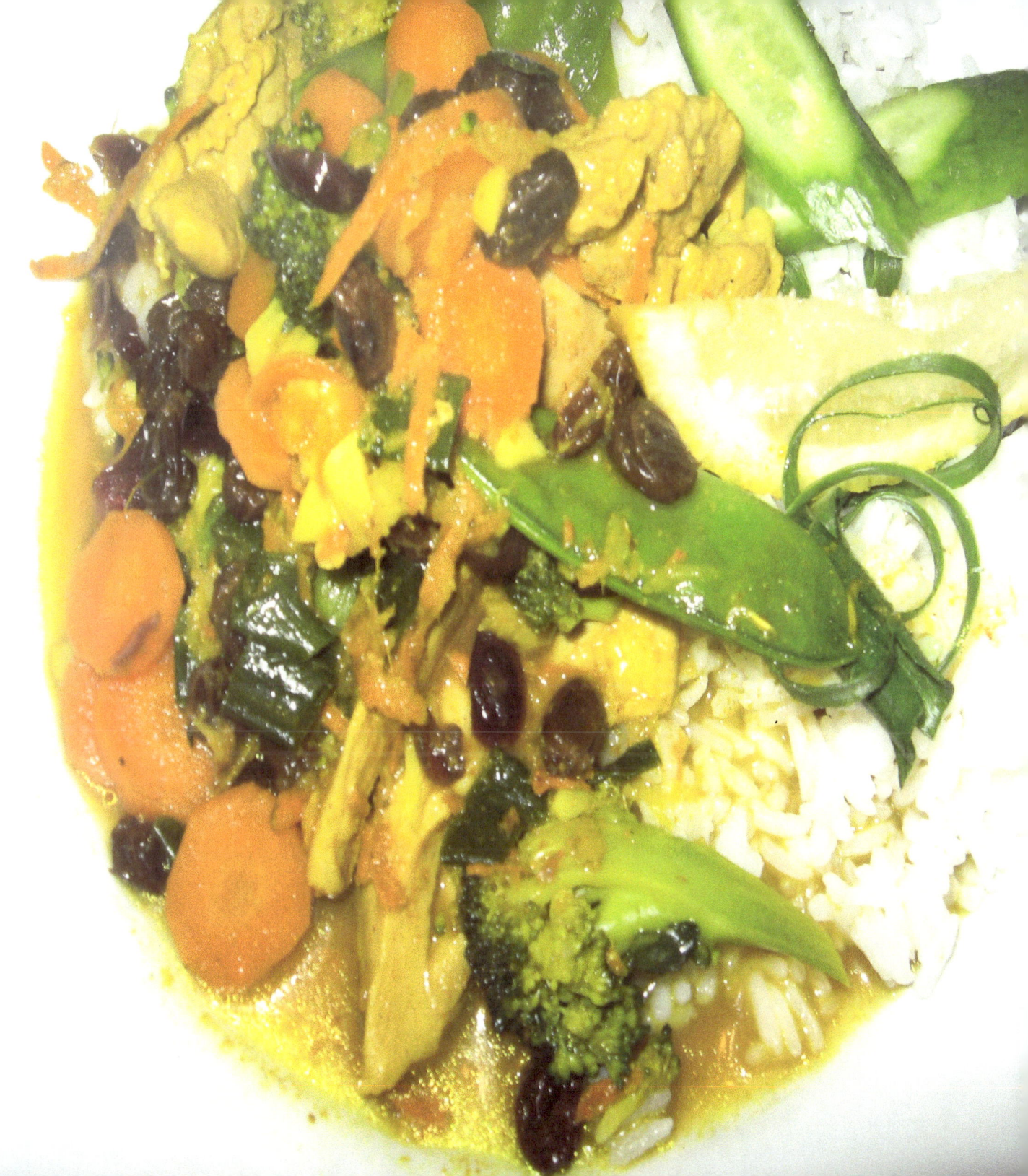

Chicken and steamed vegetables

4 pieces of tender skinless chicken fillets
2 Carrots sliced and diced
10 snow peas
3 sticks celery
2 cups of chicken stock.

Add chicken stock to small frypan
add chicken turn when cooked add more chicken stock add vegetables. A sprinkle of basil.
Add carrots sliced celery, and five minutes before you serve on rice add the snow peas.

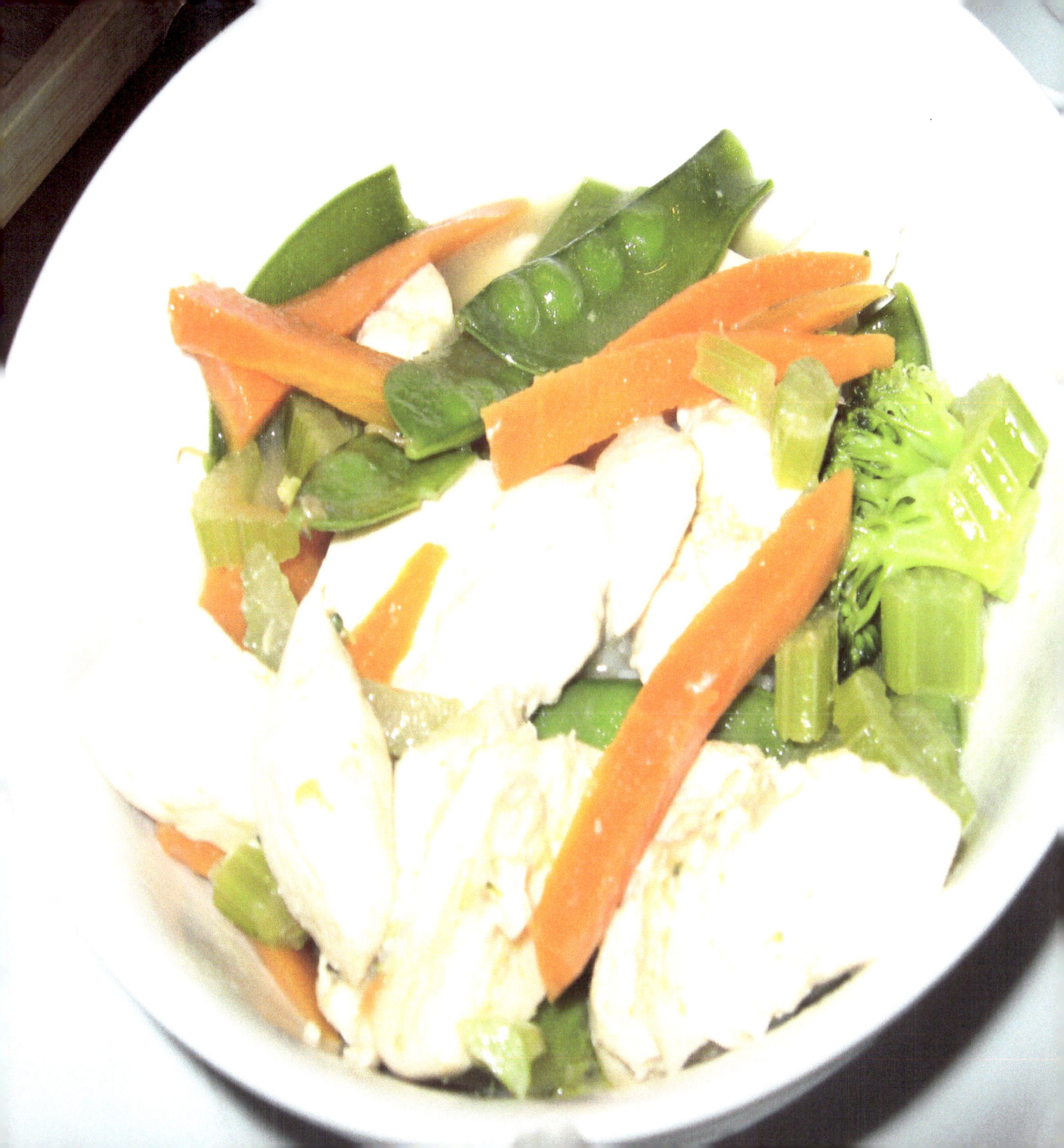

Chicken and fried rice

4 small chicken mini fillets
2 cups cooked Jasmin rice
2 sticks celery chopped
3 Jalepeno red yellow and orange slice
1 carrot thin slices
1 tablespoon a soya sauce

Coconut oil 1 tablespoon
add diced chicken cook both sides
add celery, carrots, Jalepeno sliced,

Add soya sauce stir and serve in bowl.

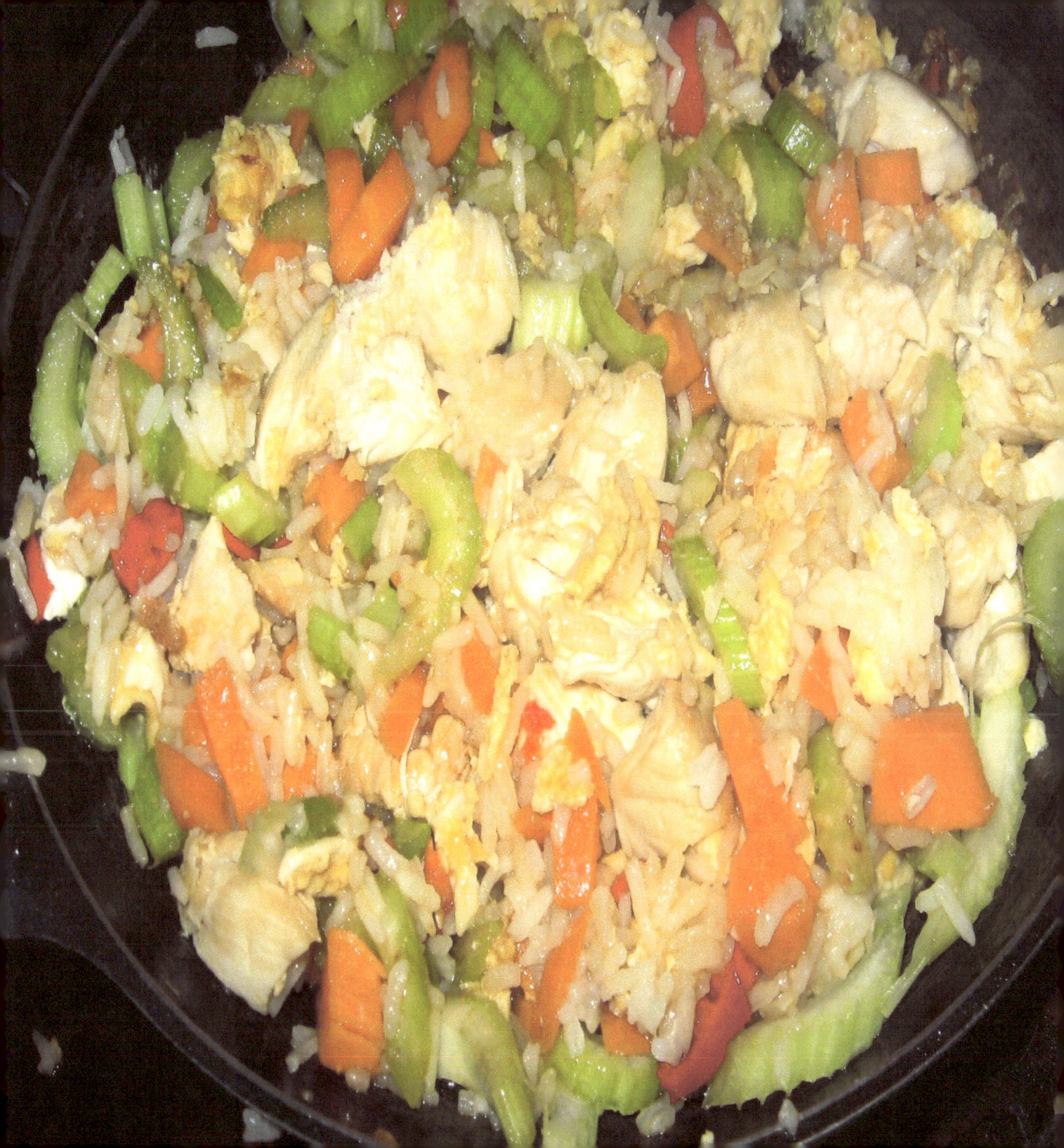

Chicken Mornay with Jalepeno

2 Cups chicken stock
4 mini chicken fillets
1/2 head of brocilli
1 zuccini sliced into thin strips
3 jalepeno sliced
1/2 tin of coconut milk light
1 soup spoon of Thai green curry

Cook chicken fillets in chicken stock turn add green curry and more chicken stock add zuccini, jalepeno, brocilli, and when cooked about 5 minutes add 1/2 tin of coconut milk lite.

serve with steamed rice.
.

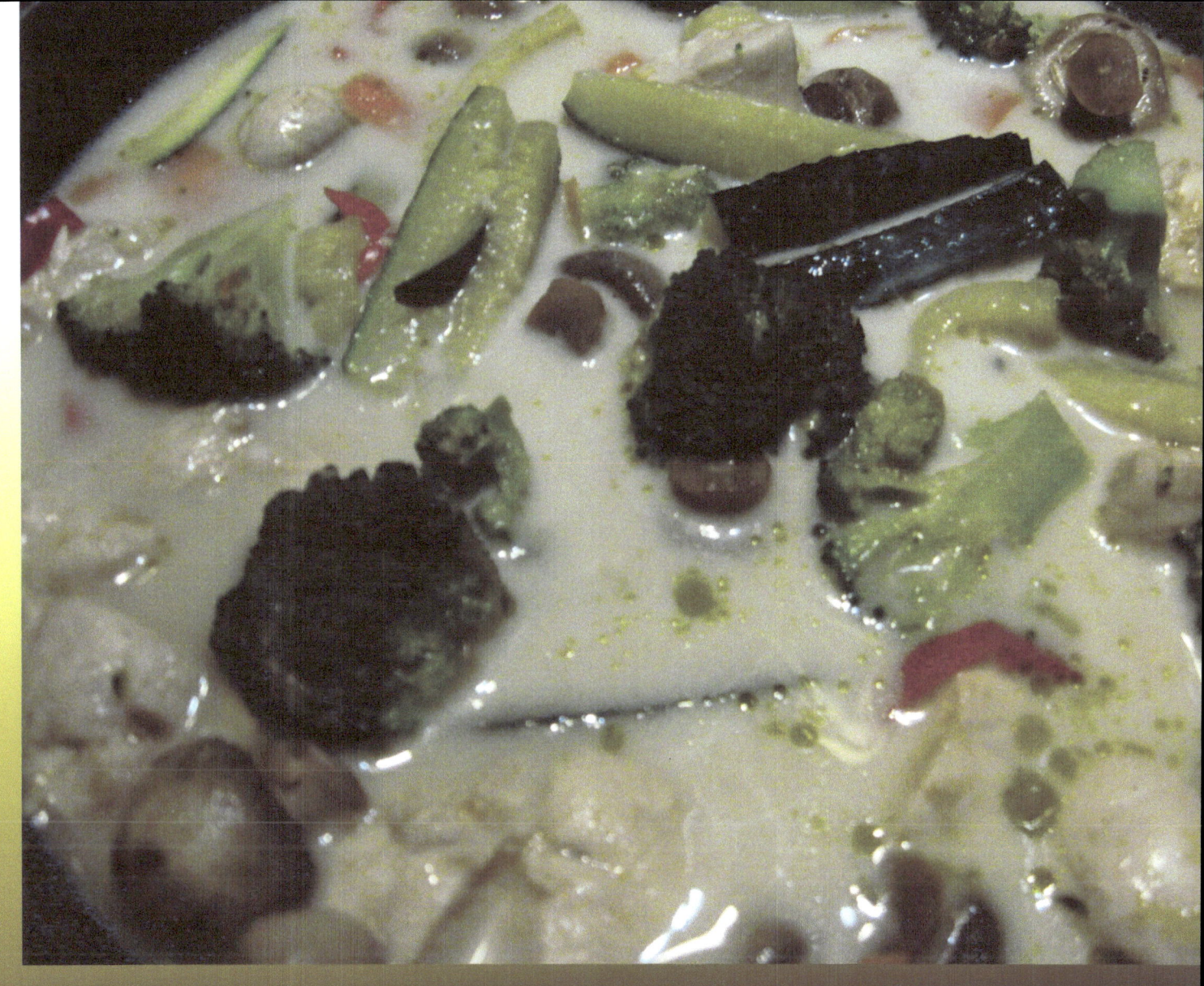

Mornay Jalapeno green curry

Chicken Thai curry

2 Cups chicken stock
4 mini chicken fillets
1/2 head of brocilli
1 zuccini sliced into thin strips
1 soup spoon of Thai green curry
6 champignons mushrooms
1 carrot sliced
8 snow peas
1/2 lactose free lite milk

Cook chicken fillets in chicken stock turn add green curry and more chicken stock add zuccini, , brocilli, and other vegetables when cooked about 5 minutes add milk.

serve with steamed rice.

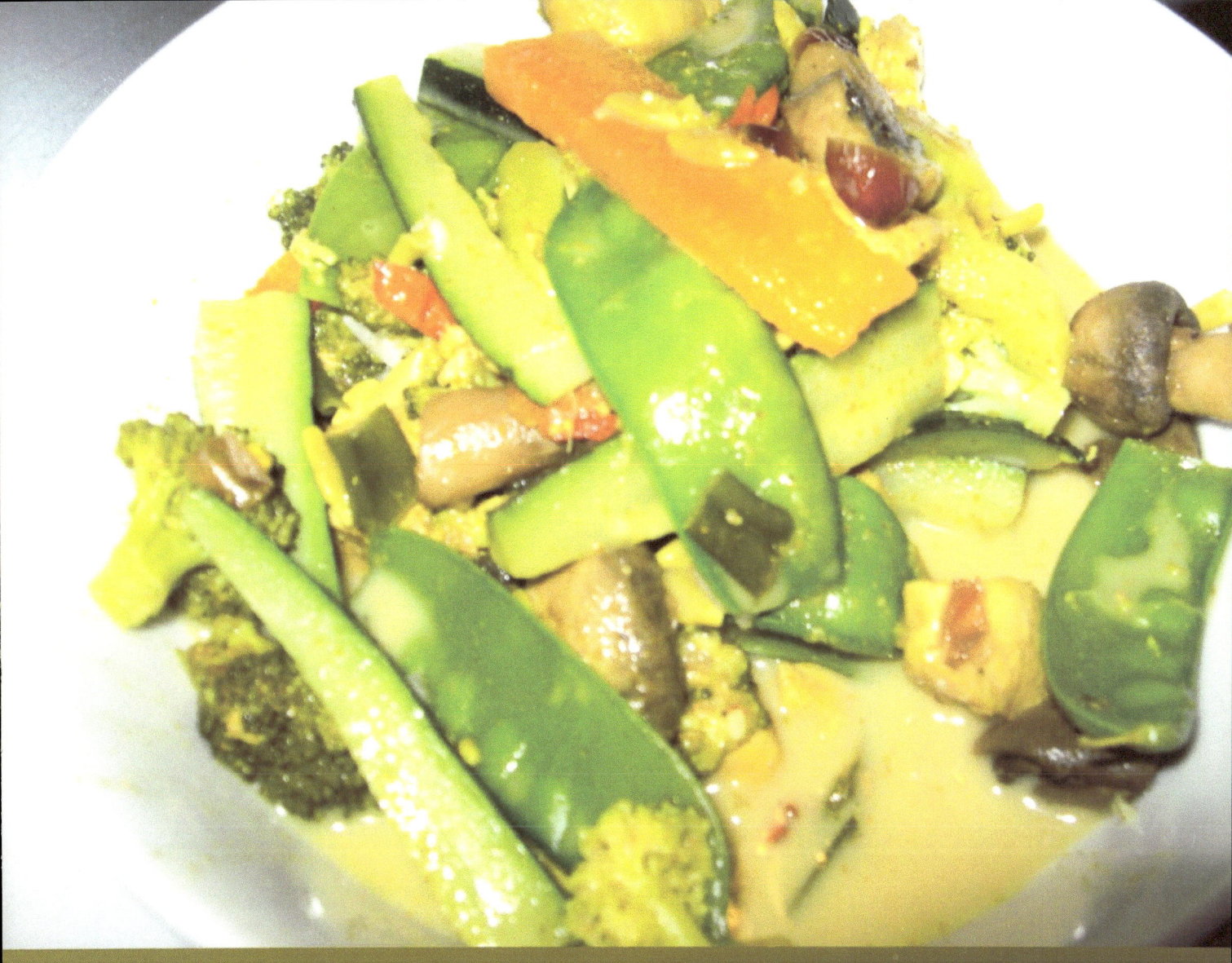
Green Thai Curry with zucchini

Chicken Indian curry

2 Cups chicken stock
4 mini chicken fillets
1/2 head of brocilli
1 cup cauliflower floretes
1 soup spoon of Clive of India curry powder
6 champignons mushrooms
8 snow peas

Cook chicken fillets in chicken stock turn
add curry and more chicken stock
add zuccini, , brocilli, and other vegetables
when cooked about 5 minutes add milk.

serve with steamed rice.

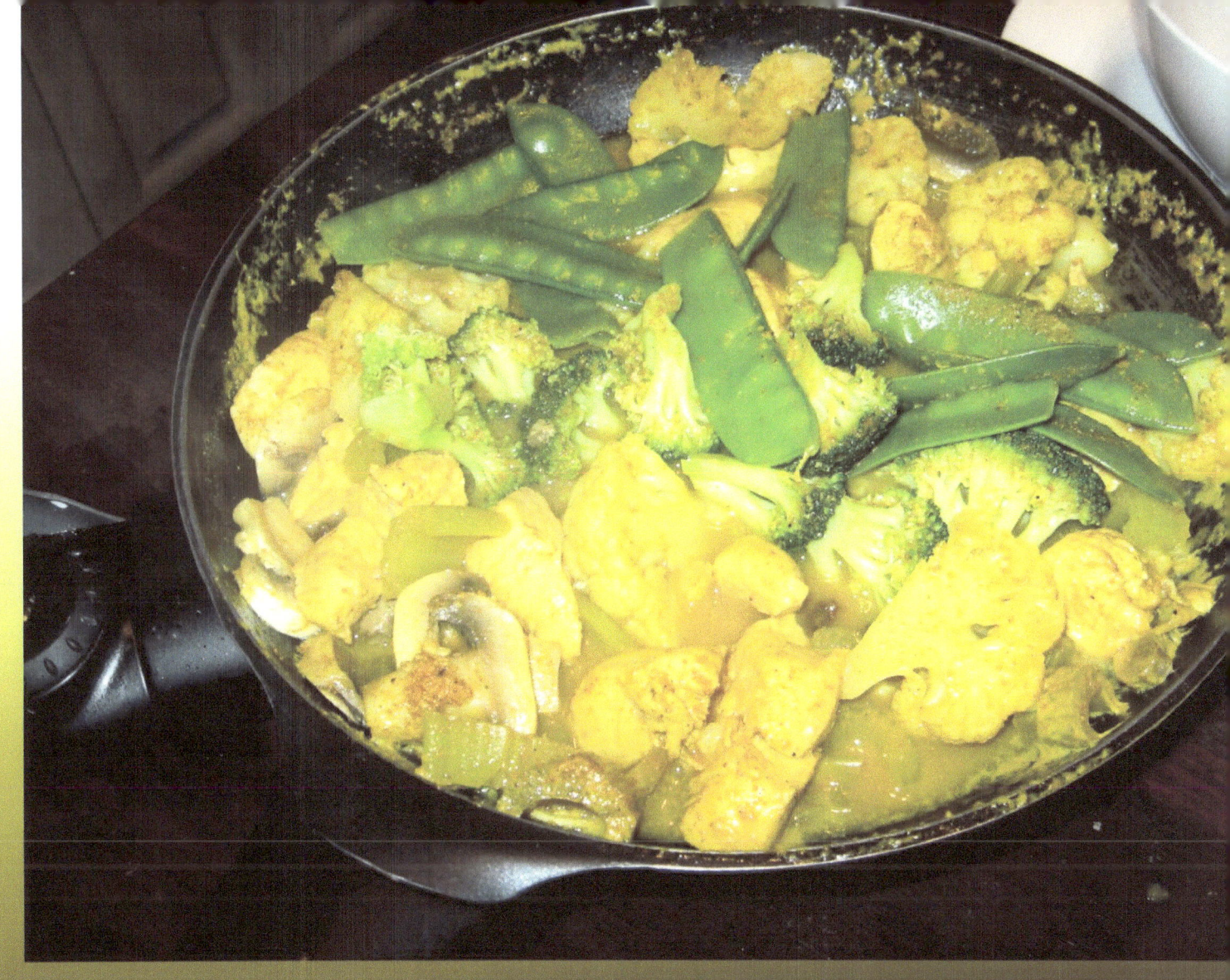

Green curry Clive of India cauliflower/ chicken

SALMON SWEET & SOUR

2 Cups chicken stock
4 mini salmon fillets
1/2 head of brocilli
1 cup celery sliced
1 cup pineapple juice
2 carrots sliced
1 zuchini sliced into long pieces

Cook salmon fillets in chicken stock turn add curry and more chicken stock
add zuccini, , brocilli, and other vegetables when cooked about 5 min add arrowroot in 1/2 cup water mixed add. Add green ginger grated to taste..

serve with steamed rice.

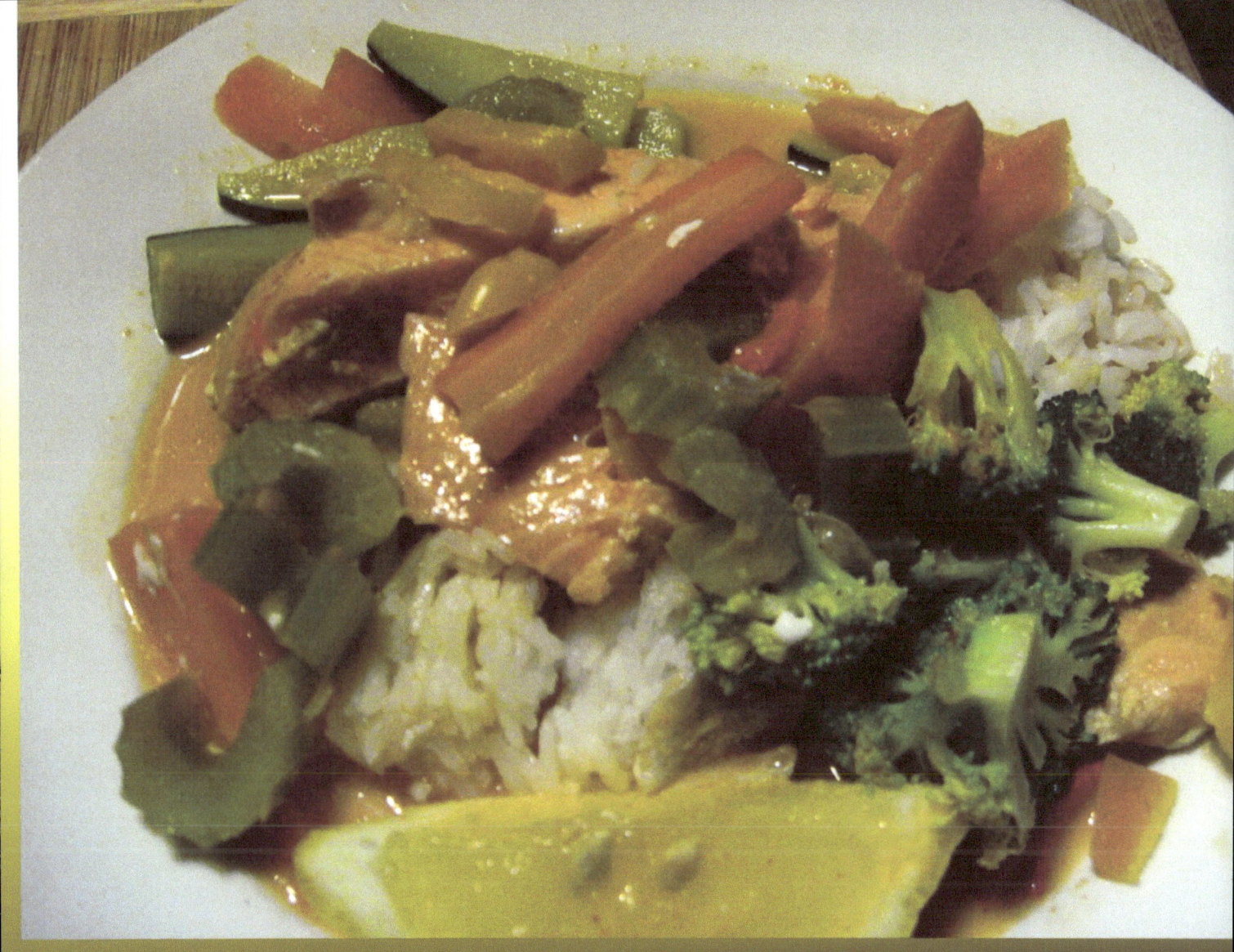

Sweet and Sour Chicken and Vegetables.

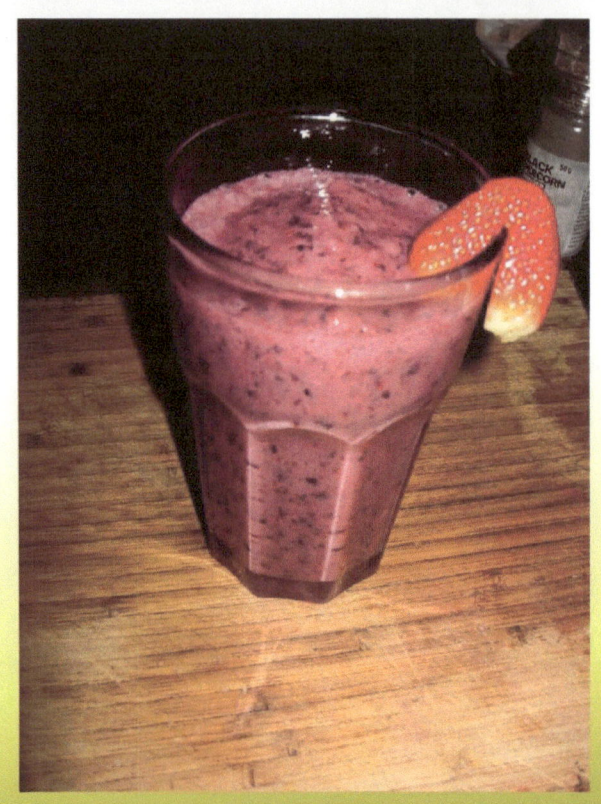

Blueberry & strawberry Frappe

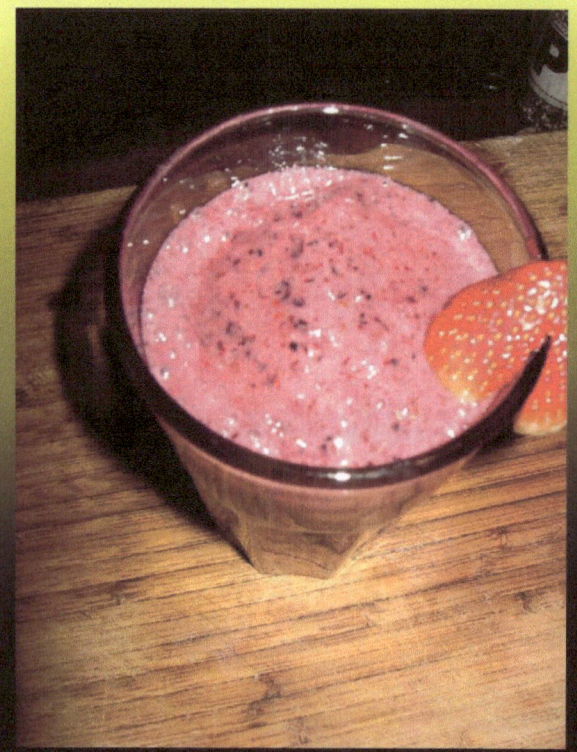

STRAWBERRY FRAPPE'

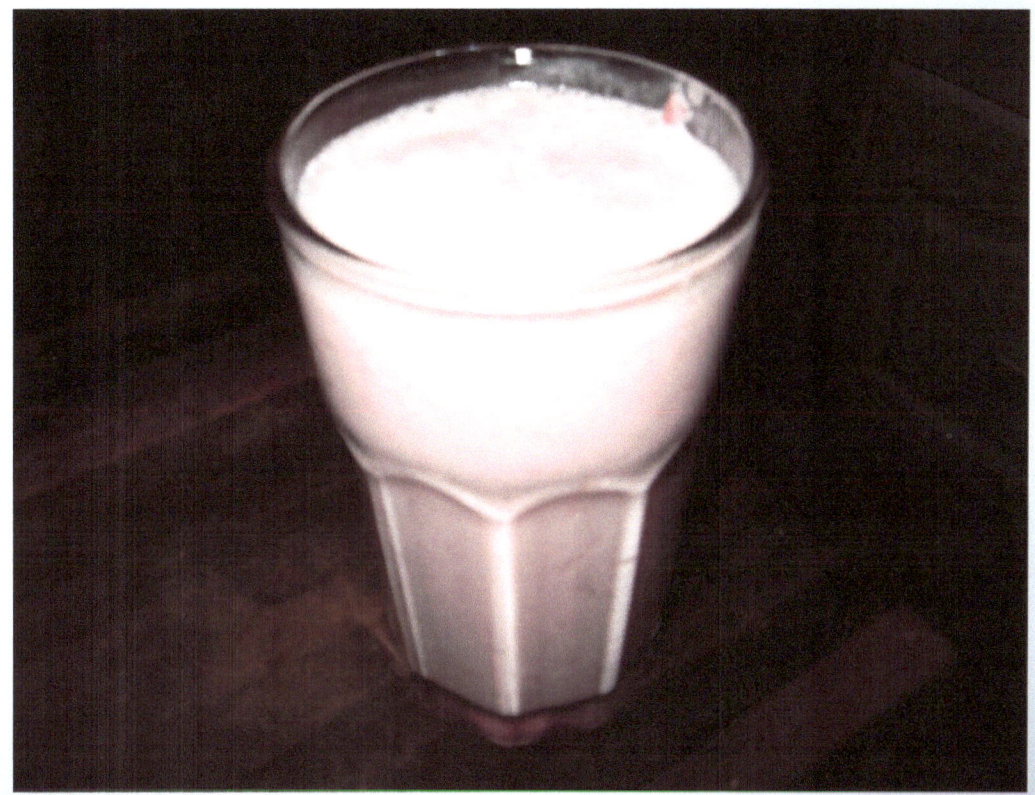

6 strawberries
1.5 cups almond milk
Mix in Blender.

www.ingramcontent.com/pod-product-compliance
Lightning Source LLC
Chambersburg PA
CBHW051819210526
45473CB00005B/1662